F

Dr. Kanu

TRAMADOL GUIDE (THIS IS AN EDUCATIONAL GUIDE AND NOT A PILL. Direction YOUR DOCTOR OR PHYSICIAN)

This game plan is utilized to help lighten moderate to enough substantial torment. Tramadol looks like opiate (sedative) analgesics. It works in the cerebrum to change how your body feels and reacts to torment.

The best procedure to utilize Tramadol HCL

Look at the Medication Guide given by your answer pro before you begin taking tramadol and each time you get a refill. On the off chance that you have any deals, ask your ruler or medication pro.

See this drug by mouth as enabled by your ruler, reliably every 4 to 6 hours as required for assistance from uneasiness. You may take this solution with or without sustenance. In the event that you have illness, it might accept this solution with sustenance. Get several information about different approaches to manage regulate diminish nausea, (for example, resting for 1 to 2 hours with as pitiable head improvement as would be sensible).

The section depends on your torment and reaction to treatment. To lessen your danger of reactions, your master may guide you to begin this remedy at a low part and constantly increment your segment. Cling to your star's course astutely. The most stunning proposed group is 400 milligrams for dependably.

On the off chance that you are more engineered than 75 years, the most outstanding suggested bundle is 300 milligrams for reliably. Make the indispensable steps not to amass your part, take the approach considerably more a significant piece of the time, or take it for a more extended time than bolstered. Truly stop the fix when so coordinated.

Torment approaches work best on the off chance that they are utilized as the central indications of torment happen.

On the off chance that you hold up until the bitterness has broadened, the cure may not work too.

In the event that you have unfaltering torment, (for example, because of joint torment), your lord may direct you to in like manner take long-acting opiate fixes. Everything considered, this drug may be utilized for abrupt (achievement) torment correspondingly as required. Other torment relievers, (for example, acetaminophen, ibuprofen) may in like way be understood. Get a few information about utilizing tramadol securely with different remedies.

This medication may cause withdrawal responses, particularly on the off chance that it has been utilized dependably for quite a while or in high zones. In such cases, withdrawal appearances, (for example, uneasiness, watering eyes, runny nose, nausea, perspiring, muscle hurts) may happen if every one of you of an unexpected quit utilizing this drug. To imagine withdrawal responses, your master may reduce your section particularly coordinated. Reprimand your position or remedy virtuoso for more subtleties, and report any withdrawal responses immediately.

Unequivocally when this arrangement is utilized for quite a while, it may not fill in too. Converse with your position if this medication quits working strikingly.

In spite of the way where that it helps different individuals, this fix may every once in a while cause dependence. This peril might be higher in the event that you have a substance use issue, (for example, abuse of or dependence on courses of action/liquor). Take this drug unequivocally as bolstered to cut down the threat of dependence. Approach your master or drug expert for more subtleties.

Tell your ruler if your anguish endures or mixes.

Reactions

Find in like way Warning area.

Queasiness, heaving, stoppage, flimsiness, bewildering, tiredness, or cerebral torment may happen. A touch of these symptoms may diminish after you have been utilizing this medicine for a long time. In the event that any of these impacts endure or increment, tell your position or prescription expert instantly.

To reject halting up, eat an eating routine taking part in fiber, drink a lot of water, and exercise. Approach your solution master for assistance with picking a diuretic, (for example, a stimulant sort with stool conditioner).

To diminish the threat of fragility and cluttering, get up particularly orchestrated when moving from a sitting or lying position.

Keep in mind that your ruler has endorsed this medication since the individual has sentenced that the unbelievable position to you is more fundamental than the threat of reactions. Different individuals utilizing this medicine don't have veritable reactions.

Tell your lord rapidly if any of these flawed yet authentic reactions happen: mental/air changes, (for example, actuating, portrayals), veritable stomach/stomach torment, take a stab at peeing, indications of your adrenal organs not working splendidly, (for example, loss of aching for, exceptional tiredness, weight rot).

Get therapeutic assistance rapidly if any of these amazing in any case seriousfainting, seizure.

This medicine may amass serotonin and basically every once in a while reason an extraordinary condition called serotonin issue/toxic quality. The danger increments on the off chance that you are other than taking different arrangements that movement serotonin, so tell your ability or remedy master of the fundamental number of fixes you take (see Drug Interactions area). Get restorative assistance in a brief instant in the event that you build up a touch of the going with manifestations: vivacious heartbeat, pipedreams, loss of coordination, authentic confusing, earth shattering sickness/heaving/division of the guts, snapping muscles, unexplained fever, strange chafing/uneasiness.

Tramadol is changed into a solid opiate medicine in your body. In express individuals, this change happens speedier and more totally than anticipated, which makes the danger of extraordinary reactions. Get therapeutic assistance rapidly in the event that you see any of the going with: moderate/shallow breathing, true laziness/have a go at blending, tumult.

A crazy inauspiciously delicate response to this medicine is brilliant. Regardless, get recuperating help rapidly in the event that you see any of the going with signs: rash, shuddering/swelling (particularly of the face/tongue/throat), super shocking, load loosening up.

This is decidedly not a hard and fast theoretical of potential reactions. In the event that you see different impacts not recorded above, contact your ruler or drug master.

In the US -

Call your master for supportive bearing about signs. You may report signs to

FDA at 1-800-FDA-1088 or at
www.fda.gov/medwatch.

In Canada - Call your ruler for
recovering enthusiasm about reactions.
You may report reactions to Health
Canada at 1-866-234-2345.

Securities

Before taking tramadol, tell your ruler or
medication ace on the off chance that
you are weak to it; or in the event that

you have some various hypersensitivities. This thing may contain lazy fixings, which can cause awfully frail responses or different issues. Talk with your medication virtuoso for more subtleties.

Prior to utilizing this medication, tell your expert or arrangement ace your remedial history, particularly of: cerebrum issue, (for example, head hurt, tumor, seizures), breathing issues, (for example, asthma, rest apnea, ceaseless obstructive pneumonic affliction COPD), kidney ailment, liver sickness, mental/viewpoint issue, (for example, perplexity, distress, vain thoughts), individual or family legacy of a substance use issue, (for example, abuse of or dependence on drugs/liquor), stomach/intestinal issues, (for example, blockage, stoppage, segment of the guts in light of sullying, debilitated ileus), take a stab at peeing, (for example, as a result of made prostate), gallbladder tainting, tribulation of the pancreas (pancreatitis), weight.

This course of action may make you questionable or moderate. Try not to drive, utilize mechanical collecting, or do any movement that requires sharpness until you are certain you can perform such exercises securely. Keep up a key detachment from mixed refreshments.

Overdose

In the event that somebody has overdosed and has veritable responses, for example, going out or have a go at breathing, give them naloxone on the off chance that open, by then call 911. On the off chance that the individual is alert and has no signs, call a deadly substance control concentrate immediately. US inhabitants can call their near underhandedness control focus at 1-800-222-1222. Canada inhabitants can call a regular unsafe substance control focus. Indications of overdose may include: moderate breathing, moderate/sporadic heartbeat, stupor like state, seizure.

Notes

Attempt not to give this reaction for different people. It is unlawful.

This prescription has been kept up for your present condition as it's been said. Attempt not to utilize it later for another condition close by at whatever point requested to do in that most remote point by your lord. A substitute fix might be essential everything considered.

Ask your lord or medicine star in the event that you ought to have naloxone open to treat opiate overdose. Demonstrate your family or family individuals the indications of an opiate overdose and how to treat it.

Missed Dose

Not fitting.

Cutoff

Store at room temperature far from light and immersion. Evade all fixes from youngsters and pets.

Endeavor not to flush meds down the latrine or void them into a channel except for at whatever guide coordinated toward do everything considered. Fittingly dispose of this thing when it is done or never again required. Course your medication master or neighborhood waste trade company.Information last changed July

Before having medicinal technique, train your position or dental pro concerning all that you use (checking master proposed drugs, nonprescription arrangements, and standard things).

A couple of kids might be reliably touchy to extraordinary reactions of tramadol, for example, absurd apathy, perplexity, or moderate/shallow/uproarious unwinding up. (See also Warning district.)

Dynamically settled grown-ups might be authentically precarious to the reactions of this medication, particularly perplexity, daze, tiredness, and moderate/shallow unwinding up.

Amidst pregnancy, this medication ought to be utilized totally when unquestionably required. It might hurt an unborn infant kid. Take a gander at the dangers and focal concentrations with your position. (Discover in like manner Warning segment.)

This strategy goes into chest milk and may once in a while effectsly influence a nursing baby kid tyke, for example, sporadic slowness, take a stab at supporting, or weight loosening up. Chest supporting while meanwhile utilizing this arrangement isn't suggested. Bearing your master before chest bracing.

Joint undertakings

Find in like way Warning zone.

Cure affiliations may change how your prescriptions work or improvement your hazard for legitimate reactions. This record does not contain all conceivable fix affiliations. Keep a synopsis of the basic number of things you use (checking drug/nonprescription meds and home made things) and offer it with your master and prescription star. Make the central steps not to begin, stop, or change the bit of any fixes without your ruler's help.

A couple of things that may interface with this game plan include: certain torment drugs (blended opiate agonist-rivals, for example, pentazocine, nalbuphine, butorphanol), naltrexone.

Taking MAO inhibitors with this fix may cause a dependable (perhaps dangerous) persistent connection. Deny taking MAO inhibitors (isocarboxazid, linezolid, methylene blue, moclobemide, phenelzine, procarbazine, rasagiline, safinamide, selegiline, tranylcypromine) amidst treatment with this strategy. Most MAO inhibitors should other than not be taken for around fourteen days before treatment with this drug. Requesting that your master when begin or quit taking this remedy.

The hazard of serotonin issue/dangerous quality improvements in the event that you are in like way taking different courses of action that development serotonin. Perspectives join road fixes, for example, MDMA/"bliss," St. John's wort, certain antidepressants (checking SSRIs, for example, fluoxetine/paroxetine, SNRIs, for example, duloxetine/venlafaxine), among others. The danger of serotonin issue/ruinous quality might be inside and out that truly matters without inquiry when you begin or advancement the bit of these cures.

Different medications can impact the arrival of tramadol from your body, which may impact how tramadol works.

Perspectives consolidate quinidine, azole antifungals, (for example, itraconazole), HIV drugs, (for example, ritonavir), macrolide counter experts harms, (for example, erythromycin), rifamycins, (for example, rifampin), drugs used to treat seizures, (for example, carbamazepine), among others.

The threat of real appearances, (for example, moderate/shallow breathing, real laziness/befuddlement) might be extended if this prescription is taken with different things that may in like way cause drowsiness or breathing issues. Tell your position or arrangement genius on the off chance that you are taking different things, for example, other opiate anguish or hack relievers, (for example, codeine, hydrocodone), liquor, cannabis, drugs for rest or trepidation, (for example, alprazolam, lorazepam, zolpidem), muscle relaxants, (for example, carisoprodol, cyclobenzaprine), or antihistamines, (for example, cetirizine, diphenhydramine).

Check the names all around of your medicines, (for example, affectability or hack and-cold things) since they may contain fixings that reason tiredness. Get a few information about utilizing those things securely.

This solution may interfere with certain examination center tests (checking amylase/lipase levels), conceivably causing false test outcomes. Accreditation investigate office staff and the majority of your experts recall you utilize this medication.

CPSIA information can be obtained
at www.ICGtesting.com
Printed in the USA
LVHW082356280619
622739LV00019B/493/P

The Ghost and
his Son

A man died leaving behind his only son of about twelve years old. As the body was being taken for cremation, the boy insisted on going with the funeral procession but his mother and others prevented him from going.

Nonetheless he stealthily went to a ridge from where he saw his deceased father was cremated. Believing that his father was residing there, he began going there at night

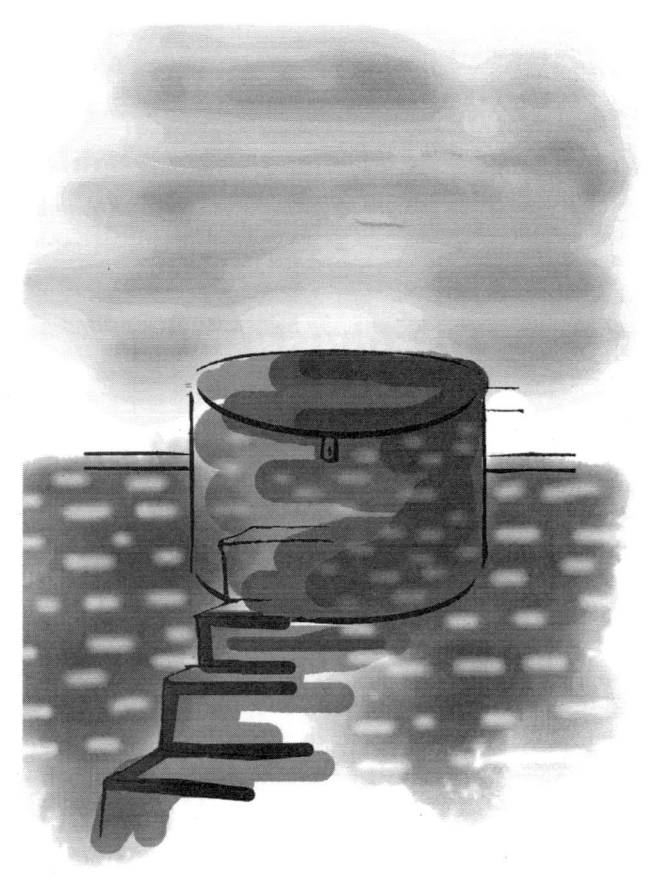

addressing repeatedly, 'Father! Father!' quite unaware his father had left this world.

One night, while calling out for his father, he saw a ghostly form. He embraced believing him to be his father and told him that before he used to be well fed and now he got nothing of the sort since he had left him.

Hearing this, the ghost pointed out to the ruined house in the neighbourhood and told him that he should dig a floor there and take the riches. He accordingly dug the floor of the ruined house and found a jar of gold coins.

The ghost never appeared to the boy again.

The Girl and
her Snake Husband

There was a man who was not satisfied with his wife. He was always angry with her. He said to himself: 'I can break a stone into two slabs, but cannot get anything from my wife; she is foolish and useless.' At last, he drove her away. She went to a field and began to live there and supported herself by begging.

One day, she found a small snake among the grasses in the field. She kept it in a basket. Next day, she found it had grown bigger and filled the basket. She then put it into a larger one but that too was filled. And so it continued to grow bigger and bigger.

She then went back to her husband's house and said to him that she had borne a snake *son* and demanded a house to raise the child. The man was afraid of the snake but was more concerned about this unusually embarrassing event that he had *a snake son*. So, he built a three-storeyed house. She put the serpent there. But the snake kept growing and filled the house too. The woman was in a fix. She had heard strange stories about snakes found in the fields. The only solution was to marry it to a girl.

She consulted with her husband. The man hesitated for a moment, thinking who would want to marry a serpent. He could not find a woman willing to marry a snake. At last he found a poor desparate widow with a daughter. He gave the widow Rs. 6,000 and took away her daughter and married her to the snake.

The girl, seeing the very large snake, wept her ill fortune. But her mother-in-law comforted her and asked her to apply oil to the snake's body. On the first night, the snake gave her a space by putting its head outside the threshold. This allowed her to sit by it and she passed the night uncomfortably.

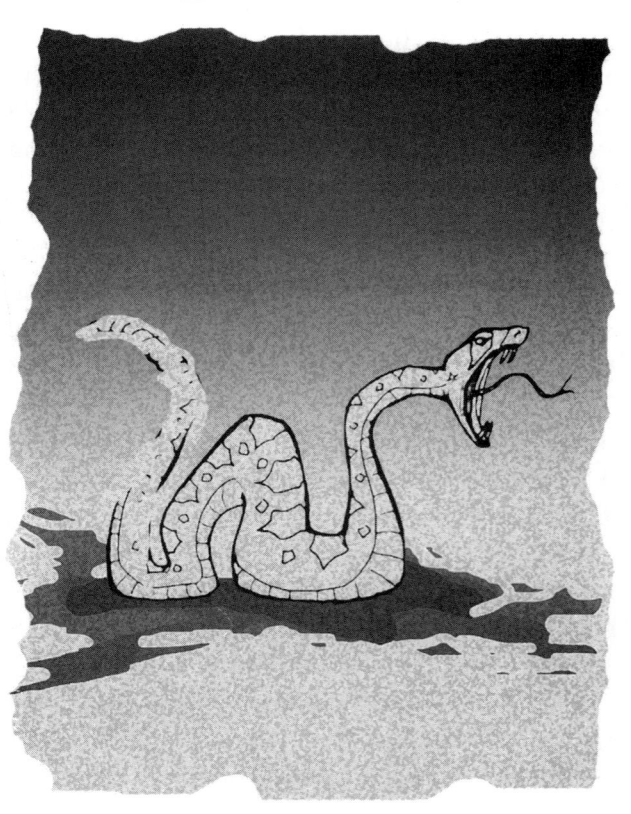

Incidently, the next day, the snake seemed to have shrunk in size. This news made the woman wonder about the tales she had heard and advised her daughter-in-law to keep applying oil on the snake's body daily. The diminishing size gave more and more space, allowing even enough place on the bed to share it. Then one day, the snake shredded off the skin and became a handsome man. She went wild with joy. But he put it back on the next morning and it became the reptile again, and she was puzzled.

She told her mother-in-law about the strange incident. She asked her daughter-in-law to burn the skin when the snake took it off. When this happened again the following night she quietly took the skin and burnt it.

Now her husband could not change back into a snake. The mother was very happy to see her son in human form and her daughter-in-law was filled with joy at the turn of her fortune.

It is said that a treasure buried in the ground becomes a snake, and the snake if kept by human beings turns into a man.

13

The Boy and
the Demoness

There was a demoness who transformed into a pretty young woman and appeared before a well-off man. The man found her very beautiful and wanted to marry her even though he already had four wives. She agreed to marry him.

In the first night, she killed and ate one of his wives. In the second night she did the same with the secomd wife and in the following night the third one was killed and eaten up.

The fourth wife, suspecting something unusual about the disappearances of fellow co-wives, ran away to a neighbour's house with her fourteen-year old son.

She and her son plotted to find a way to expose her husband's evil new wife. She told her son:

'Your father's new wife must have a hand in the sudden disappearances of your step-mothers. We must devise a plan. If I tell your father, he will not believe me. He is completely under her spell. He will rather rebuke and kill me.'

The son began thinking of ways to get rid of his new step-mother. He went to town and met an old woman who was intimate with his step-mother. She often went to the old woman to have lice removed from her hair and for gossip. The boy offered her two gold coins for information about her friend.

During their next meeting, the old woman, in the course of their chit-chat, casually asked her about her life. She revealed that she was the daughter of a powerful demon and that her soul lived in an island across seven seas. There was a large *pipal* tree with many parrots living on its many branches. On top of that tree was a nest and a large parrot, in whose body her soul resided.

The old woman told the secret to the boy in exchange for two gold coins. The boy was now in a dilemma as how to cross the seven seas to catch the parrot. Once more, the boy went to the old woman to find out how this could be done for which he was willing to pay four more gold coins.

The next time the demoness went to town, the old woman slyly told her that she should be careful and not reveal the method by which the seas are crossed. The demoness, not aware that she was giving away her secret, replied that she had a pair of sandals, by which the seas can be crossed, carefully locked in a box and that box was always underneath her bed.

On getting this invaluable information, the boy went to his father's house disguised as a fakir. There he begged for alms and also requested to be put up for the night. Since no one risks offending an ascetic, he was lodged in a room previously occupied by his mother.

At midnight, taking advantage of demoness' absence from the room, he quietly removed the sandal from the box from under the bed. He put them on his feet and crossed the seven seas. He found the large *pipal* tree with many branches, inhabitated by many parrots. He carefully climbed the tree and caught the large parrot in

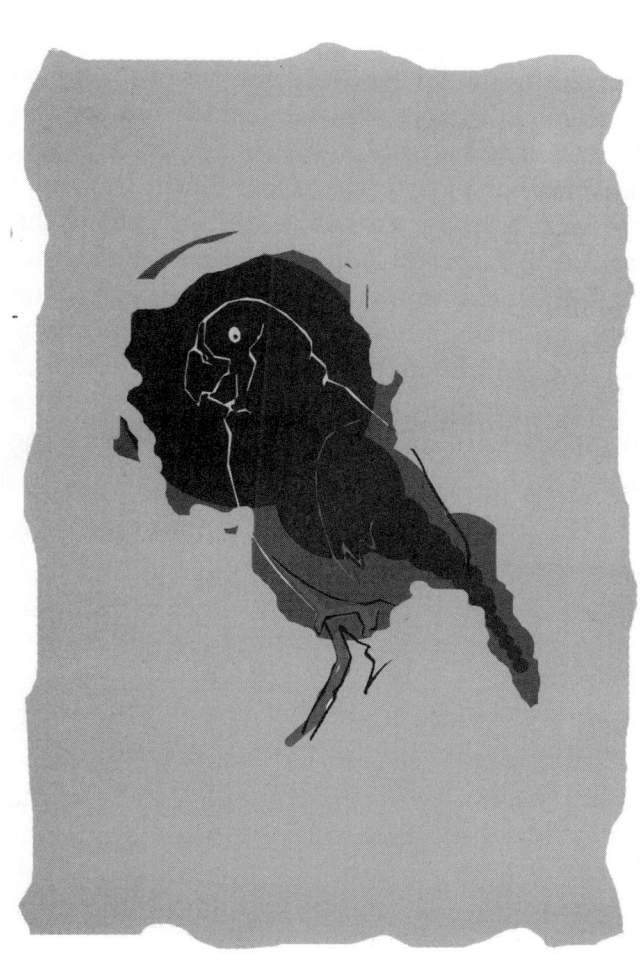

the nest at the top. He then crossed back the seas and appeared before his father's house.

By then the demoness had felt the uneasiness and when she came out of the house with her husband, she was horrified to see the parrot, with her soul inside, in the boy's hands. Despite her plea to spare her life in exchange for large fortune, the boy cut off the head of the parrot in front of them and other people who had gathered to see what was going on. The demoness thereupon died, bringing normalcy to the neighbourhood. Earlier, people had noticed strange unexplained incidents, like disappearances of some of their livestocks since the man had brought in his fifth wife.